# THE MAGIC OF NATURAL GLP-1

## *LOSING WEIGHT WITHOUT INJECTIONS*

BY:
M.D. WELLS

Covenant Freelance Services
Green Valley, Arizona

The Magic of Natural GLP-1

Losing Weight Without Injections



ISBN: 978-0-9706661-2-3

First edition 2026
Printed in the United States of America
Cover Image: Covenant Freelance Services via Canva.com

Medical Disclaimer: M.D. Wells is not a health care practitioner. ALL information in this book is purely for informational and educational purposes. If you have any questions, please do your own research or consult with your healthcare practitioner.

Publisher:
Covenant Freelance Services
472 N. Ramos Lane
Green Valley, AZ  85614
USA

# DEDICATION

This book is dedicated to:

All of my girlfriends
who have battled weight over the years!

We’ve connected with this saying:
"Brain cells die,
Skin cells die,
Even hair cells die.
But fat cells... must have accepted Jesus Christ as their Lord and Savior
because they seem to have eternal life".

# CONTENTS

# PREFACE

## The GLP-1 Revolution

The rise of GLP-1 drugs has been nothing short of miraculous. In medical trials they have produced results rivaling bariatric surgery. Initially developed for Type-2 diabetics, their stunning side effect was significant weight loss. Further studies developed dosing specifically for weight loss on severely obese patients. These drugs act on the brain and gut to reduce hunger and food cravings.

The surprising fact is their development from natural GLP-1 produced in the gut. These drugs simulate natural GLP-1 but in higher, longer lasting doses. They also come with side effects; and in many cases, significant financial burden. The question is, can you boost natural GLP-1, losing weight without the side effects and disadvantages.

The answer is 'yes.' Even those who are prescribed a GLP-1 drug are advised that they work best when paired with a healthy diet and regular physical activity, not as a replacement for them. The reality of weight loss is that it is a lifelong commitment. Fat cells have "epigenetic memory." They retain markers from past obesity promoting rapid weight regain. This is especially true in rapid weight loss as provided by simulated GLP-1 drugs. There are no quick fixes. Fat cell memory is stubborn but can be managed by sustained weight loss for a prolonged period. Cell turnover can take up to ten years.

Learning how to manage weight naturally is the key to long-term success.

This book is not intended as a replacement for medication in diabetics or in the management of severely obese people. However, they can certainly complement a more effective management of obesity and diabetes with the principles in this book.

This book is designed for the average adult struggling with those few extra pounds. Studies reveal 35% to 49% of the American population attempt to lose weight annually. Yet, the average Body Mass Index (BMI) of Americans continues to rise. Since the body is programmed to defend against loss of fat, the "yo-yo" effect continues to plague us. The key to sustained weight loss is knowledge of how the body processes the foods we eat.

This is not a recipe book nor a food plan. It contains food-based strategies to boost GLP-1, improve metabolism and manage hunger without injections. It focuses on understanding how the body produces GLP-1 naturally and offers sustainable weight loss habits.

Your journey of GLP-1 knowledge begins here.

# *THE JOURNEY BEGINS*

# CHAPTER ONE

# WHAT ARE GLP(s)?

GLP stands for glucagon-like peptide. These are hormones our body produces primarily in the intestinal tract. Their job is to regulate blood sugar. When you eat, specialized cells in your gut release these peptides into your bloodstream. Each GLP has different functions.

## GLP-1

This is the most well-known member of the family. It is a 30-amino acid peptide hormone. When you eat, L-cells in your small intestine release it into the bloodstream. This triggers the pancreas to increase insulin secretion. Insulin allows glucose (sugar) from food to enter cells to be used for energy. It also stabilizes blood sugar by enabling storage of any excess glucose in the liver, muscles and fat cells. This prevents hyperglycemia. Simultaneously, it notifies the pancreas to suppress glucagon secretion. This prevents the liver from releasing stored glucose. It also slows how quickly the stomach empties. This slowed movement of food from the stomach into the small intestine signals the brain it is full. You feel full faster and longer. As a result, you eat less.

## GLP-2

Glucagon-like peptide-2 is another gut-derived hormone. It is a gut health specialist. This 33-amino acid peptide hormone focuses on promoting intestinal growth, repair, and nutrient absorption. It also slows stomach emptying, allowing more time for nutrient absorption and triggering the brain that it is full. It promotes growth and repair of the intestinal lining (mucosa). It aids in increasing the height of the intestinal finger-like projections that absorb nutrients. It increases blood flow to the intestines supporting optimal digestive function. GLP-2 also strengthens the intestinal barrier, reducing intestinal permeability (leaky gut). This protects against harmful substances entering the bloodstream. In addition, GLP-2 reduces inflammation in the intestinal tract and promotes healing of damaged tissue.

Synthetic GLP-2 (like Teduglutide) is used for treating patients with shortened bowels due to surgical removal. They are also being studied for Crohn's disease, inflammatory bowel disease, ulcerative colitis and malabsorption issues.

## GLP-3

This remains the most mysterious member of the family. It has had limited research but is now gaining traction. It appears to play a role in metabolic regulation. This means it controls cellular chemical reactions to balance nutrient intake and energy demand. GLP-3 activates glucagon receptors, which can increase thermogenesis (energy/calorie burn).

Synthetic GLP-3 may be the new generation of weight-loss drugs. Eli Lilly is conducting Phase 3 clinical trials for Retatrutide. It is designed as a triple hormone agonist (targeting

GLP-1, GIP, and glucagon receptors). It is showing results in reducing appetite, lowering blood sugar and increasing energy expenditure.

# CHAPTER TWO

# HISTORY OF SYNTHETIC GLP-1

Since people with Type 2 diabetes have a reduced or impaired response to natural GLP-1, scientists began experimenting with development of a medication which could mimic its effects in the body. In the mid 1980s, John Eng was studying bioactive peptides from the venom of the Gila monster. He identified a peptide named Exendin-4 which stimulated insulin secretion in rodents. He collaborated with Amylin Pharmaceutical (AstraZeneca) to begin a series of clinical trials. It was shown to be highly significant in lowering HbA1c in Type 2 diabetic patients. As a result, Exenatide was approved for treatment of diabetes in 2004. Exenatide was marketed as Byetta in 2005. Byetta required twice daily injections.

In 2010 Novo Nordisk introduced Victoza as a once daily injectable GLP-1. This was later approved for weight management under the name Saxenda. In 2017 Novo Nordisk revolutionized the market with semaglutide, a once weekly form, marketed as Ozempic for glycemic control in Type-2 diabetics. During clinical trials, semaglutide was noted to have contributed to weight loss. New clinical trials were initiated for Wegovy, the identical semaglutide but with different dosing. It was approved by the FDA for chronic weight management in 2021.

These drugs are known as receptor agonists. An agonist mimics a natural substance binding to a cell receptor, triggering a biological response. In 2022, Eli Lilly introduced Tirzepatide, a dual agonist (GLP-1 and GIP). GIP stands for glucose-dependent insulinotropic polypeptide. These hormones are secreted in response to food intake. They regulate metabolism and appetite. This combination is found to be more effective than GLP-1 alone. It was marketed as Mounjaro for Type-2 Diabetes and as Zepbound for dosing in weight loss management in 2023.

Investigations are ongoing with companies investigating oral versions of these medications. Novo Nordisk has marketed Rybelsus (oral semaglutide) for type 2 diabetes. Eli Lilly has marketed Foundayo, an oral GLP-1 for weight loss.

Remember, these synthetic drugs are designed to mimic naturally occurring glucagon-like peptides. These synthetic drugs can be life saving for metabolic disorders like diabetes. Using them for weight loss is secondary. Natural foods can also boost GLP-1. I believe there is a healthier option for weight loss while simultaneously reducing any potential side effects.

# CHAPTER THREE

# DISADVANTAGES OF SYNTHETIC GLP-1

**Prescription Only**

- Physician care is required.
- Baseline testing prior to prescription: kidney function, liver health and lipase level. Lipase is a digestive enzyme, produced by the pancreas, to breaks down dietary fats (triglycerides) for absorption. High levels in the blood often indicate pancreatic damage.
- Monthly checkups while dosing is increased helps manage dose dependent side effects like nausea and diarrhea.
- Lab monitoring every 3 to 6 months to evaluate metabolic makers, weight loss progress, kidney function and potential severe side effects.

**Cost**

- These drugs often exceed $900 to $1400 per month.
- Insurance coverage is often limited for weight loss. Approximately half of GLP-1 users discontinue treatment due to cost.

## Counterfeit GLP-1

Due to the high cost of pharmaceutical GLP-1 drugs, unscrupulous suppliers are creating counterfeit, unregulated versions to exploit the high demand. Instead of highly controlled processes used for pharmaceutical grade products, these are produced with unverified chemical ingredients, not FDA approved. They are packaged in pens designed to look like legitimate products. They are sometimes labeled as “custom-mixed” or “generic.” The raw materials often come from China and are then shipped elsewhere for packaging and distribution. The counterfeit pens often contain incorrect labeling, misspellings, or name the ingredient rather than the brand name.

Unfortunately, some weight loss clinics, spas, and online pharmacies sell “compounded” products which are actually fake. Some fake pens have been found to contain harmful, inactive or lower-grade ingredients than genuine medication. Compounded versions are not reviewed by the FDA for safety or efficacy. These products may vary in potency (too strong or too weak) and have the potential for risk of contamination when not sourced from a reputable, licensed pharmacy. Compounded semaglutide should only be used if prescribed by a healthcare professional and filled by a reputable, state-licensed compounding pharmacy.

## Common Side Effects

- Nausea (common initially)
- Vomiting
- Diarrhea or constipation
- Reduced appetite

- Headache
- Fatigue
- Injection site reactions
- Potential pancreatitis (rare)
- In addition, research indicates 25%-39% of total weight loss can come from lean muscle mass. The more muscle you lose, the fewer calories your body can burn naturally. This contributes to rapid weight gain once the synthetic GLP-1 is discontinued. Loss of muscle mass also contributes to frailty and physical instability.

**Serious But Rare Side Effects**

- Pancreatitis
- Gallbladder problems
- Kidney issues
- Thyroid tumors (in animal studies)

**Contraindications**

- Personal or family history of medullary thyroid cancer
- Multiple endocrine neoplasia syndrome type 2
- Severe gastrointestinal disease

# CHAPTER FOUR

# TRIGGERING NATURAL HORMONES

Skip the expensive injections and lose weight naturally. The good news is that research verifies certain foods can trigger natural production of GLP-1. In some studies, participants have lost an average of 10%-15% of their body weight over a year. Yes, it takes time. Remember, rapid weight loss contributes to a high percentage of reduction in muscle mass. As natural GLP-1 is boosted over time, a steady, gradual loss of weight helps insure a higher percentage of true lost fat rather than muscle. Even a 5%-10% reduction in body weight can lower blood pressure, improve metabolic health and decrease the risk of certain conditions like fatty liver disease.

GLP-1 drugs help weight loss by making you feel full on less food, decrease appetite, and reduce cravings for junk food. Long before these drugs, dietitians recommended foods to help patients lose weight and keep it off. The science behind these foods reveals their ability to impact hunger in the same ways. These include leptin, ghrelin, cholecystokinin (CCK) and peptide YY. Foods high in protein, fiber and healthy fats can trigger the release of GLP-1 hormones.

## Leptin

Leptin is a hormone produced by fat cells, often called the "satiety hormone." It regulates long-term energy. Leptin signals the brain when the body has sufficient energy stores, reducing hunger and promoting energy expenditure. Hens produce this hormone in their liver and scientists have found it in both the yolk and white of eggs. Certain foods can increase leptin sensitivity helping the brain recognize 'fullness.' These include healthy fats like olive oil, nuts, seeds, and avocados which are high in omega-3 fats. These fats are anti-inflammatory. This is key, as inflammation blocks leptin signaling. Foods like garlic, onions, asparagus, and leeks also reduce inflammation in the gut. Lean meats like fish, chicken and turkey reduce triglycerides, improving leptin sensitivity. Alternately, high-saturated fat and refined carbohydrates in processed foods contribute to leptin resistance. Don't bother taking leptin supplements if your body is resistant. Eat foods known to increase sensitivity.

## Ghrelin

Ghrelin is a hormone produced in the stomach which tells the brain you are hungry. Levels of this "hunger hormone" rise as the stomach gets empty. Eggs and quinoa are known to suppress ghrelin. You can also reduce the ghrelin response by eating smaller meals on a more regular basis. Eating six small meals per day is much better than three large meals. Scientists have also found poor sleep as a contributor to high ghrelin production. Aim to get seven to eight hours of high quality sleep each day.

## Cholecystokinin (CCK)

CCK is a hormone produced in the small intestine. When fats and proteins enter the first part of the small intestine (duodenum), CCK is released to stimulate gallbladder bile and pancreatic enzymes. These rush to break down food for absorption. In fact 'cholecystokinin' means to 'move the gallbladder.' CCK also suppresses stomach emptying until the first batch is done to maximize absorption. Indirectly this suppresses your appetite by telling the brain your stomach is full. CCK also triggers muscle contractions enabling food to move along through your intestines. Certain food are key CCK triggers. Long-chain fatty acids are potent stimulators. Known as LCFAs, these contain 13-21 carbon atoms and are crucial dietary lipids.

LCFAs are found in salmon, mackerel, walnuts, almonds, flaxseed, avocados, olive oil, soybean oil, dairy fat and animal fats. In addition, lauric acid (C12) is a saturated medium-chain fatty acid that increases CCK release up to five-fold. Its highest concentration is found in coconut oil. Protein rich foods trigger CCK release. When losing weight, strive for the lean proteins in fish, chicken, eggs, yogurt, cottage cheese, and mozzarella. A whey protein shake will also deliver. The fiber in beans also increase CCK response. Last but not least, coffee has long been recognized as a stimulant for gallbladder emptying which is driven by CCK. Maybe that after dinner coffee should be considered.

## Peptide YY

Pancreatic peptide YY is a hormone secreted in the small intestine. There are two forms of PYY containing between 34 and 36 amino acids. It is released in proportion to caloric intake. PYY is secreted along side of GLP-1. It is a key signal to reduce appetite and food intake. It peaks 1-2 hours after eating. Again, it is mainly stimulated by ingestion of fat and protein. Carbohydrates break down into glucose and do not activate receptors on intestinal L-cells in the same way. Carbs are absorbed higher up in the digestive tract. PYY is released from the lower small intestine and colon. The high insulin response from carbohydrates leads to faster return of hunger compared to meals high in protein. Due to its ability to suppress appetite, PYY is being studied for potential treatments of obesity. In addition to the foods mentioned in CCK release, leafy greens, whole grains (oats, barley) and berries also contribute to PYY response.

It should also be noted that fermented foods, like yogurt, kefir, sauerkraut, and kimchi help to support a healthy intestinal microbiome. A healthy gut boosts the release of all the satiety hormones.

# CHAPTER FIVE

# NATURAL GLP-1 FOODS

**Salmon, Sardines, Mackrel & Trout**

The high quality protein and omega-3 fats in these high-fat fish are strong natural triggers to produce and release GLP-1 in the intestinal tract. In addition, they may protect pancreatic cells. Fish also ranks among top foods in terms of making you feel full and satisfied. Slower digestion also tempers blood sugar levels.

**Legumes: beans, lentils, chickpeas**

Legumes are rich in nutrients and very filling. They achieve the goal of slowing digestion due to their high protein and fiber content. Slower digestion leaves more food in the stomach making you feel fuller. It also tempers blood sugar levels reducing cravings. Lentils actually came in highest on this list. One cup contains 18 grams of protein and 15 grams of fiber. This is generally more protein and fiber than most people eat in an entire day. Black beans also have 15 grams of fiber and only slightly less protein. One cup of cooked chickpeas (garbanzo beans) typically contains 14.5 grams of protein and 9 grams of fiber.

**Oats**

Oats are high in a soluble fiber called beta-glucan. Studies show beta-glucan increases satiety and enhances GLP-1 secretion. As an added bonus, oats help reverse insulin resistance and lower LDL-cholesterol levels.

**Edamame**

Edamame are immature soybeans harvested before they fully mature. They are often found in Asian cuisine and have a slightly sweet, nutty, buttery taste. One cup of cooked edamame contains approximately 18 grams of protein and 8 grams of fiber. They also contain healthy fat and are rich in iron, potassium and magnesium.

**Peanut butter**

Peanuts are a good source of plant-based protein and fiber. Both monounsaturated and polyunsaturated fats support GLP-1 response without causing digestive discomfort. Use natural peanut butter without added sugars or hydrogenated oils. Portion control is advised due to its high calorie density. Try peanut butter on whole grain toast to maximize fiber.

**Whey Protein Shakes**

A whey protein shake will stimulate natural GLP-1 release. It's an excellent choice prior to a meal to improve glucose response and reduce hunger. Whey protein often outperforms or matches other protein sources for satiety. When whey is combined with calcium or other healthy fats in meals, it can maximize GLP-1 release.

**Greek Yogurt**

Traditional Greek yogurt is strained so it has twice the protein of regular yogurt. It also contains less than half the sugar making it a healthier choice. Traditional Greek yogurt contains both high protein and calcium. Protein is one of the strongest stimulators of GLP-1. Calcium works in tandem with protein to further increase GLP-1 production. As a fermented food supporting gut microbiota, it combats against natural GLP-1 resistance.

**Eggs**

Eggs are considered a powerhouse for stimulating GLP-1. As a high-quality protein and healthy fat source, they directly boost the body's natural production of GLP-1 leading to increased fullness and reduced appetite. Research has shown that a high protein breakfast combined with high healthy fats, such as eggs, reduces food intake over 24 hours. Research has also found that egg consumption lowers the 'hunger' hormone ghrelin.

**Barley**

Barley is a great source of high soluble fiber. Barley is a nutty grain which can be boiled and eaten in place of pasta or rice. It contains beta-glucans which inhibits fat cell growth, and is known to increase GLP-1 levels. In studies, animals fed barley extracts lowered body weight gain and visceral fat gains. Visceral fat is located deep within the abdomen surrounding vital organs. It is dangerous because it releases inflammatory compounds and fatty acids directly into the liver. This drives chronic inflammation and insulin resistance. Overall, barley produces an anti-obesity effect.

**Quinoa**

Quinoa is considered a complete protein, containing all nine essential amino acids. It is also high in fiber. Because of its low glycemic index, it stabilizes blood sugar suppressing the release of ghrelin, the hunger hormone. Simultaneously, it supports a gradual increase in GLP-1 levels.

# CHAPTER 6

# GLP-1 STIMULATING SNACKS

Feeling a little hungry? Snack on these healthy GLP-1 boosting alternatives. Minimize sugary snacks, refined carbs and greasy fast foods. These cause blood sugar spikes forcing the pancreas to produce excessive insulin. Over time it increases the risk of insulin resistance and weight gain. Insulin resistance can often be reversed or significantly improved with the correct diet, exercise and improved sleep. The secret to success is fiber, healthy fats and protein. This triple threat is the secret to satiety and weight management which begins with hormone management. Stimulating the GLP-1 hormone is the key.

**Nuts**

Pistachios, almonds, walnuts and pecans contain fiber, plant-based protein, and healthy fats that trigger significant GLP-1 release. Walnuts have the highest amount of omega-3 fatty acids which build cell membranes and reduce inflammation. Because of calories, limit your snack to about a quarter of a cup.

### Sacha Inchi

Known as the Inca peanut, this seed is native to the Amazon rainforest. It is considered a superfood because it is rich in protein, antioxidants and high levels of omega-3, 6 & 9 fatty acids as well as vitamins A & E. Omega-3s are known to enhance leptin sensitivity helping to reduce cravings. It acts as a natural DPP-4 inhibitor enhancing the body's ability to lower blood sugar and increase GLP-1 and GIP. The seeds are sold roasted and make a great addition to trail mix. Sacha Inchi oil can be used in salad dressings. It increases HDL (good cholesterol) and reduces LDL (bad cholesterol). The seeds can also be ground and used as protein powder in smoothies.

### Peanut Butter

Peanuts are rich in both monounsaturated and polyunsaturated fats. Studies show these help increase natural GLP-1 levels in the blood. They are also high in fiber and protein making you feel fuller longer. Be sure to select natural peanut butter without the added sugars or hydrogenated oils. Because peanuts are calorie dense, peanut butter should be used in moderation. Pair it with another fiber-rich food like celery or whole-grain crackers to enhance GLP-1 response.

### Hummus and Veggies

Chickpeas contain a unique type of fermentable fiber. This is broken down in the colon to produce short-chain fatty acids which are the main energy source of colon cells. This strengthens the gut barrier and helps regulate metabolism. Hummus is made with chickpeas and tahini (sesame seed paste). Pair hummus with vegetables high in water and fiber content like bell peppers, cucumbers, celery, snap peas, and raw broccoli or cauliflower florets. For quick homemade hummus recipe, see the recipe offer at the end of this book.

**Avocado**

Avocados are also high in monounsaturated fats and fiber triggering GLP-1. Slowed digestion leads to prolonged feelings of fullness and reduced appetite. Adding a healthy avocado snack can help manage hunger and support steady energy levels throughout the day. Try avocado toast or make an avocado salsa. A recipe for avocado hummus is also included in the free offer at the end of this book. Enjoy it with the vegetables listed above.

**Chia Seeds**

Chia seeds are another complete protein containing all nine essential amino acids. The nine essential amino acids cannot be produced in the body and must be obtained through diet. Foods that contain all nine are considered 'super foods.' Chia seeds are also packed with soluble fiber. Two tablespoons of chia seeds contain 11 grams of soluble fiber. Soluble fiber dissolves in water to form a gel-like substance in your stomach and intestines. This slows digestion prolonging a feeling of fullness and enhances the release of GLP-1. The high omega-3 content of chia seeds also helps manage blood sugar levels.

**Dark Chocolate**

The flavanols in cocoa beans are full of anti-inflammatory agents and antioxidants. The beans contain stearic acid, an anti-inflammatory saturated fat. However, unlike animal fat, it does not increase bad cholesterol. The human body does need some saturated fat for lipid metabolism and cell membrane integrity. The recommended amount is 10% of daily calories.

There is a difference in chocolate. Milk chocolate is only about 30-50% cocoa (cocoa solids and cocoa butter), sugar, and the addition of milk solids. White chocolate contains cocoa butter and milk solids but no cocoa solids. Dark chocolate contains 50-90% cocoa (cocoa solids and cocoa butter), sugar and sometimes vanilla. To garner all the health benefits, choose organic dark chocolate of at least 80%.

Dark chocolate also contains resveratrol, a strong antioxidant with many cardiovascular benefits such as blood pressure and brain health. It is also high in magnesium, a mineral supporting the nervous system as well as sleep and relaxation.

# CHAPTER SEVEN

# FUTURE RESEARCH

Stanford University medicine researchers used artificial intelligence to find a new weight-loss peptide. The new molecule, labeled BRP, is naturally occurring and led to weight loss in mice and pigs. It also worked without some of the common side effects of semaglutide (Ozempic) such as nausea, constipation and loss of muscle mass.

## The Gut-Brain Connection

Our body possess a bidirectional communication network. The central nervous system consists of the brain and spinal cord. It receives sensory information from the body, interprets it, and sends out instructions on how to react. The enteric nervous system is a mesh-like network of approximately 500 million neurons. These neurons are embedded in the lining of the gastrointestinal tract. It is actually capable of controlling digestive function independently of the brain and is often called the "second brain." These two systems communicate via the vagus nerve. Also known as the tenth cranial nerve, it is the longest nerve in the autonomic nervous system. It controls involuntary functions like heart rate, breathing, immunity and, you guessed it, digestion. Because of this intricate connection, mental stress can cause digestive issues. Conversely, gastrointestinal issues can affect mood and brain function.

## GLP-1 Verses BRP

GLP-1 functions primarily in the gut and pancreas, also sending signals to the brain. BRP works through an entirely separate pathway. BRP acts specifically in the hypothalamus, which controls appetite and metabolism. The hypothalamus is the body's main control center. It is a region within the brain roughly the size of a pea. Small but powerful, it has many functions. It acts as the body's thermostat, regulates water balance and nutrients. It also controls hormone release, sexual drive and reproduction, thyroid function, and coordinates fight or flight responses. Among many other things, it plays a key role in emotions, behavior and motivation including the regulation of mood influencing hormones.

BRP directly influences brain circuits which control appetite and metabolism. It enhances lipid oxidation, leading to increased fat burning while not causing unpredictable swings in blood sugar levels. BRP is a small peptide made up of just 12 amino acids. The Stanford researchers compared it with GLP-1 on neuronal cells which transmit information. GLP-1 had a threefold effect while BRP had a tenfold effect. Injections of BRP show promising results in weight loss due almost entirely to loss of fat. The mice also had improved glucose and insulin tolerance. The positive results were achieved without the common side effects of GLP-1s. Clinical trials in humans will hopefully begin soon.

## Natural BRP

BRP is newly discovered and current literature does not provide information on natural triggers. We do know, however, that it is a peptide made up of 12 amino acids. As we discussed in chapter six, there are nine essential amino acids your body is unable to produce on its own. They must be obtained through foods. Foods that contain all nine are considered 'super foods.' Top sources include lean beef, poultry, eggs, fish, milk, cheese, yogurt, whey protein, soy (tofu, tempeh, edamame), quinoa, buckwheat, chia seeds, and spirulina. Other foods when combined, like beans and rice, will also provide all nine essential amino acids. When we give our bodies the correct fuel, we can be sure, it will produce the necessary building blocks for health and well being.

# CHAPTER EIGHT

# A HOLISTIC APPROACH TO WEIGHT LOSS

Many factors play into a successful natural weight loss program. The more of these factors you can apply, the better the outcome.

## Sleep Quality

Sleep quality is vital to weight loss. Poor sleep sets you up for making very bad decisions. The brain's frontal lobe is responsible for decision making and impulse control. Lack of sleep impairs it, causing reduced metabolism, slower activity, reduced focus, impaired working memory, lower impulse control and decreased creativity. You'll probably skip exercise because you're too tired. You'll be too tired to make dinner and choose take-out instead. When you're over tired, the brain's reward center kicks in. It starts looking for something that 'feels good' like that slice of cake. Studies have shown that lack of sleep causes people to choose high carb snacks and twice as much fat as those who slept at least eight hours. So, a sleepy brain not only craves the wrong foods, but lacks the impulse control to say 'no.'

Cortisol spikes are triggered with too little sleep. This is a stress hormone signaling your body to conserve energy. When cortisol levels rise, your body holds on to fat, refusing to burn it for fuel. Diminished sleep also causes insulin resistance. It hinders your body's metabolic ability to process insulin properly. Insulin is the hormone needed to change sugar, starches, and other food into energy. If not converted, it is stored as fat. Studies have shown a 30% reduction in insulin sensitivity in as little as four days of insufficient sleep. Consider sleep like nutrition for the brain. Strive for between seven and nine hours each night.

If you have trouble sleeping, don't work in the bedroom. Train your brain that the bedroom is for relaxation (not entertainment) and sleep. Shut down your computer, cell phone, and TV at least one hour before going to bed. Take a warm bath, meditate or read a book. Avoid caffeine at least five hours before bedtime. Turn out the lights. Darkness cues your body to release melatonin, a natural sleep hormone. Stick to a schedule, even on weekends.

**Water**

Water is present in every cell in our bodies. Around 60% of the human body is water. The lungs themselves are approximately 83% water. The brain and heart around 73%. It is essential for good health. Water increases metabolism aiding the body in burning fat. Studies have shown that even mild dehydration can slow down metabolic rate by 3%. A few glasses of water in the morning will help you wake up.

When you drink water between meals, it helps you feel full, reducing cravings. Oftentimes, the body perceives thirst as hunger. Staying hydrated helps break down food so the body can absorb nutrients. During weight loss, water helps to rid the body of waste and metabolized fat. It flushes out sodium (salt) reducing water retention. The kidneys and liver are better able to flush out toxins. In addition, it increases blood flow to the muscles reducing muscle fatigue while helping electrolyte balance. This translates to quicker recovery during exercise.

## Alcohol

There are several reasons why alcohol inhibits weight loss. It is possible to lose weight while drinking alcohol, but it is much harder to do. If you are unable or unwilling to eliminate it entirely, try reducing it as much as possible.

- The body treats alcohol as a toxin. It will, therefore, stop the fat burning process in order to prioritize the toxin metabolization and removal.
- Alcohol can disrupt sleep cycles contributing to the issues listed above under sleep quality.
- Alcohol is very high in empty calories. It provides no essential nutrients nor any trigger for GLP-1.
- Alcohol stimulates the same brain signals as during starvation leading to increased appetite.
- Alcohol contributes to dehydration, loss of electrolytes and increased inflammation. Loss of electrolytes creates a craving for salty, high-carb foods.
- When alcohol is consumed before a meal, it has the ability to make food taste better, leading to overeating.
- Psychologically, it lowers inhibitions, leading to poor food choices and overeating.

## Exercise

Exercise can be difficult for many people. Begin with mild exercise if necessary. Consistency is the key. A brisk walk is a good way to expend energy without extreme exertion. Even if weight loss is minor, consistent mild exercise has the ability to increase muscle mass and reduce fat around the internal organs. Short bursts of high intensity exercise, with brief rest periods in between, is very effective in burning maximum calories. It can also boost metabolism for an entire day after a workout. Weight lifting builds muscle. The more muscle you build, the greater your resting metabolic rate. Your body burns calories to maintain muscle mass. In other words, you will burn more calories doing nothing. Due to the risk of muscle injury, it is best to consult a trainer prior to beginning a weight lifting program.

Running, jogging and cycling are all good ways to burn excess calories. One exercise, swimming, gives you a full body benefit. It leverages the high resistance of water to build muscle and burn calories. It is also excellent for joint health. For consistency, the best exercises are the ones you enjoy. Aim for about three hours of moderate-intensity exercise per week plus strength training on two or three days.

## Limit Carbs

When carbohydrates are consumed, the digestive process breaks them down into glucose (simple sugar). As it is absorbed into the blood stream, it raises blood sugar levels triggering the pancreas to release insulin. This hormone allows glucose from the bloodstream to enter cells where its used for energy. Carbs, in an of themselves, are not bad. In fact we need them. Glucose provides energy to the organs, muscles and nervous system. In fact, glucose is the brain's only source of fuel. If you experience symptoms of low blood sugar (shaking, sweating, chills, dizziness, rapid heart beat, confusion) eat carbohydrates and sugar to bring blood sugar levels back to normal.

Insulin regulates blood sugar levels, preventing them from becoming too high (hyperglycemia). Symptoms of hyperglycemia include increased thirst, blurred vision, frequent urination and headaches. Insulin also promotes storage of excess glucose in the liver, muscles and fat tissue. When we eat too many carbohydrates, not balanced by fiber, fat and protein, it leads to higher releases of insulin. High release over long periods of time, leads to insulin resistance. The body's cells fail to respond to insulin making it difficult for glucose to enter cells. Blood sugar levels rise leading to pre-diabetes and weight gain. It also causes you to feel hungry all the time no matter how much you eat. Eat carbs in moderation and incorporate them with proteins, fats and fiber. By reducing the overall glucose burden, the body's cells may become more sensitive and responsive to insulin, improving natural sugar-regulating mechanisms.

## Avoid Highly Processed Foods

Ultra processed foods are formulations of preservatives, emulsifiers, sweeteners and artificial colors with little to no food value. They are engineered for overconsumption. Easy to eat, they are digested rapidly before the gut can signal the brain that it is full. The formulation is designed to trigger the release of dopamine, the brain's 'feel good' hormone. The reaction is similar to addictive substances. These foods have also been linked to increased risk of cardiovascular disease, high blood pressure, cancer, dementia, and higher mortality rates. The main sources are sugary drinks, packaged snacks, ready-to-eat meals, processed meats, spreads and sauces, and instant items like soups, noodles, toaster pastries and even granola bars. You'll go a long way toward your goal, by eliminating highly processed foods.

**Kick-Start Your Day**

Begin your morning with fiber rich foods. This sets the tone for balanced blood sugar levels throughout the day. Try peanut butter on whole wheat toast, overnight oaks with chia seeds, Greek yogurt with chia seeds, or blend some berries or chia seeds in a whey protein shake. Add a booster drink, like green tea with breakfast.

**Snacks & Meals**

Choose snacks with fiber, protein and healthy fats. Even small servings will keep hunger at bay between meals. Include avocados and omega-3 rich foods into your meals. Meals should include a combination of lean protein or plant-based protein, high quality fiber and healthy fats. Salmon is the top choice in omega-3 and protein. As previously stated, this triple threat is the secret to satiety and weight management, stimulating the GLP-1 hormone.

* * * * *

While medications offer significant, rapid, weight loss, they are accompanied with many potential side effects. Let's be honest. It's not possible to boost natural GLP-1 levels to the same therapeutic levels achieved by medications. These medications maintain high hormone levels for days. In addition to side effects, their greatest detriment is caused when you have to stop them. Very rapid weight gain can result especially due to loss of muscle mass.

Natural stimulation due to diet and lifestyle changes works gently over time. It is healthier for your body, carries virtually no side effects, reduces loss of muscle mass and is much lower cost. Following the holistic approach trains you for a consistent life-long journey of weight management as well as a strong, healthy body.

This book is aimed at achieving natural weight loss, not treating underlying diseases. If you have underlying health conditions like diabetes, it is always recommended to consult with a healthcare professional before making significant changes. Medications are often necessary for managing certain medical conditions.

Take the information you have learned in this book and create your own daily meal plan from the suggested foods you enjoy. Get a good nights sleep. Drink plenty of water. Add a little exercise and you are on your way to a successful, healthy, natural GLP-1 weight loss program.

# ABOUT THE AUTHOR

M.D. Wells spent over forty years involved in the medical profession. Before retiring she was the Program Manager for a Vascular Fellowship Program. Having assisted in training future vascular surgeons, she understands the necessity of following 'doctor's orders.' Her experience in medical research has aided her in compiling this book and in her own weight-loss journey. She holds a degree in Business Administration.

---

## How to Order

The Magic of GLP-1

*Losing Weight Without Injections*

Paperback or Ebook

Available on Amazon.com

If you have enjoyed this book, help others by submitting a positive review on Amazon.

---

# ADDITIONAL TITLES

## By M.D. Wells

### *Colon Procedure Recipes*
### *Low Fiber—Low Residue Meals*

Are you undergoing a colon procedure? A different set of nutritional rules apply during colon procedures. The doctors may give you a single sheet of DOs and DON'Ts, but nothing really useful. They use terms like soft diet, low-fiber diet, and low-residue diet. What does it all mean? Better yet, have you tried to find tasty recipes meeting their criteria?

When the author's husband was scheduled for a colonoscopy, followed by a colon resection, she knew a special diet was required. She wanted to ensure the best possible outcome. Her experience in medical research aided her in compiling this handy reference and recipe guide. Compiled from her own recipes, this makes the process easier and more enjoyable. Some of the recipes are so good, you'll want to keep them even after you get back to 'normal.'

**What You'll Find Inside**

- The difference between low fiber, low residue and soft diets
- DOs and DON'Ts of food choices
- Easy to digest foods to promote healing
- Recipes meeting the doctor's criteria
- Meal suggestions for breakfast, lunch, dinner and snacks

**Available as Paperback on Amazon.com**

Paperback: ISBN #978-0-9706661-3-0

# ***FREE OFFER***

Join the email list for future offers and receive a free recipe PDF, *Two great GLP-1 Boosting Snacks.*

Easy Homemade Hummus

Avocado Hummus

To get your free recipes:

Email: m.d.wells.usa@gmail.com

Put "Join" in the subject line. In the email body, tell us where you obtained this book.

* * * * *

If you have enjoyed this book, help others by submitting a positive review on Amazon.

Made in the USA
Monee, IL
04 November 2026

67387915R00026